Cancer Glue for Energy

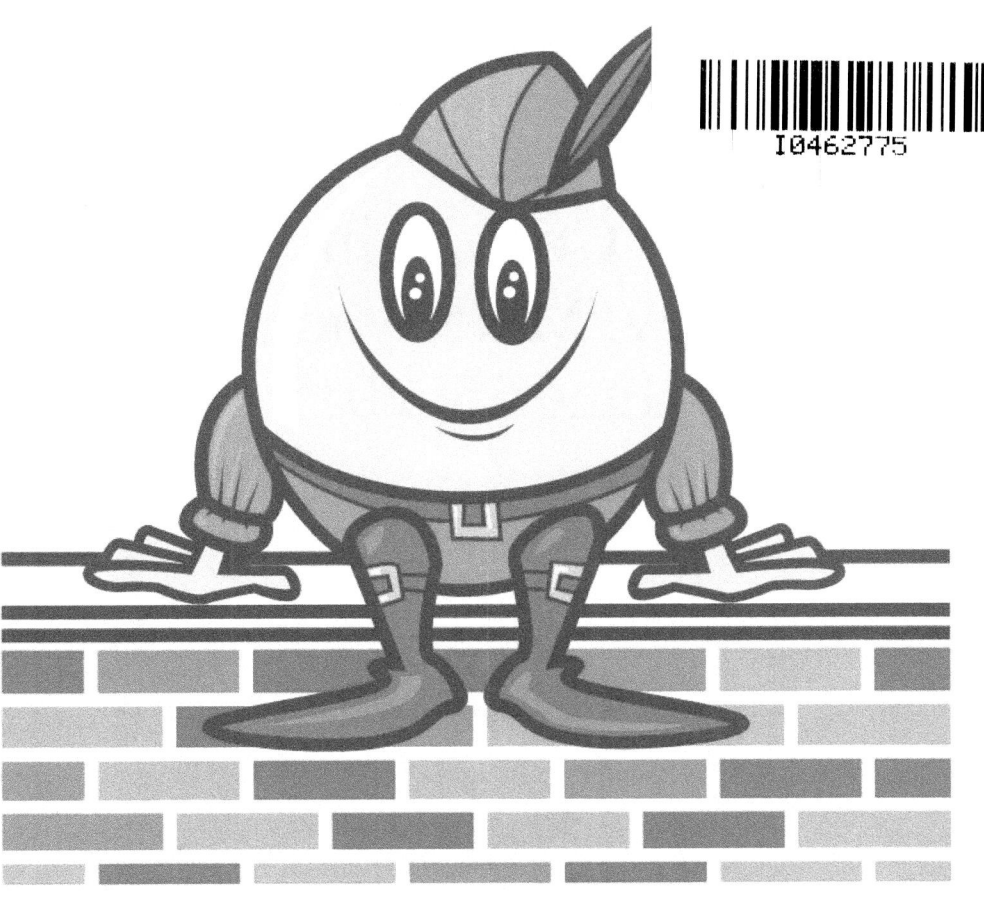

Consider Pranic Healing To Clean, and Enhance Your Energy!

Reverend Mike Wanner

Copyright
Rev. Mike Wanner
June 15, 2019

Selected Images Used by License

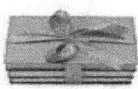

Introduction

When I was a child, my father got sick with cancer, and he had a hard time, and eventually, God called him, and I missed him. That was many years ago, and I wished that I could have done more for him.

I did not understand, but I wanted to, and it was impossible to know what to do to help others. I tried to comprehend but could not find answers.

The wanting to understand has influenced my life. The one thing that I remembered so firmly was the importance of kindness.

While the hospital situation back then was very complicated, I was helped tremendously by the kindness of the ambulance crews that came and soothed my father as they did the tough job of making him as comfortable as possible.

The ambulance organization that moved him is Burholme First Aid Corps Inc., and their motto was "Not For Self, But For Others."

When I came back from the United States Air Force after serving in Vietnam, I joined the volunteer organization and, now, forty plus years later, I still volunteer to help others.

In 2015 I wrote a book about Burholme, "Emergency Medical Kindness in the Cradle Of Liberty: Big City - Cracked Bell" as that year the Pennsylvania Dept of Health and the PEHSC named them The Best EMS Agency in Pennsylvania.

Dedication

I dedicate this book to the patients in Cancer treatment, and their Healing Arts care teams, including all Credentialed Caregivers of Medicine, Psychological and Psychiatric Professionals, Faith-based counselors, and Complementary Care Providers.

Practitioners and Master-Teachers of the spiritual healing modalities are excellent facilitators who help to balance and soothe the active components of the emotional and mental and spiritual crises of cancer survivors. I have talked about the Reiki, and the Integrated Energy Therapy® (IET) modalities extensively in earlier *"Cancer Glue For"* Series books and would like to expand on "Spiritual Healing," "Energy Healing," "Faith Healing." "Laying On Of Hands," "Energy Medicine" here.

Prana seems to allow more than subtle energy sharing. It appears to be an adaptive access way to effectively clear, smooth, filter, reconfigure, and discharge harmful or disruptive energy and refresh healing stimulation.

Table of Contents

1 - What is Prana

Prana is the life force that flows through all human beings, and it is pivotal to healing. The Human energy inside all of us is called subtle energy, which is a natural energy that is different than the Alternating Current and Direct Current energy that we see in our houses, vehicles, and batteries.

I taught Reiki (The Usui System of Natural Healing) for many years and a delightful and effective way to demonstrate subtle energy was two people holding hands and then holding a subtle energy sensitive ball which would light up when both parties touched it and completed the circuit that had the ball light up.

I have introduced Prana in earlier Cancer Glue Books and ways to nurture it. Love from Kids and Reiki and Family Energy and Miracles and Dowsing Power are all helpful.

Nurturing the energy of Cancer patients is of optimal importance to me as that is the single most significant deficiency that I have heard from patients – "I don't have any energy."

Unfortunately, too many people have that expectation which assures a struggle that is not helpful. Correcting that is recommended.

A simple energy concept is that "Energy follows Thought" so that expecting high energy and believing it is already present sets patients up for success in their struggle to heal.

2 - Why I am Writing This Book

I have moved towards support in as many ways as I can. I write a lot about healing, and my ministry of healing messages continues to come full circle.

I received some training at Cancer Treatment Center of Philadelphia and learned some more about what is possible to help those in the struggle of cancer.

With this book, I would like to share with the world some things that I have discovered so they can help soothe more people and set them up for success.

One thing that I have heard most over the years is that the patients have no energy.

To me, talking about that can exacerbate the problem. I encourage better ideas that focus on finding energy through:
1. Positive Thinking
2. Meditation
3. Mindfulness
4. Sensitivity to others needs
5. Self-determination
6. Asking Doctors for Energy Advice
7. Nutritional Awareness

3 - Disclaimer

I, the author, am not involved with clinical cancer care, but I have talked to many cancer patients during decades of pre-hospital ambulance care and transportation and also many years of Hospital Pastoral Care. I am sharing what is coming to me to spread understanding and trigger conversation that can be helpful. It may be that the discussion needs finessing, and I invite your wisdom into the mix.

My guidance has suggested that a lot can be done to soothe the times for cancer patients and their families. I will detail my views which are not the expert positions of a Cancer Center Clinician or technician or social worker, or Medical Practitioner or Psychologist or Psychiatrist or another expert who might be helpful here.

I have said, everything about cancer may seem very complicated, but there are always practical and straightforward ideas that you can embrace when a person is open to see common sense items that are within their capability. Please be diligent and check with attending nurses and physicians before doing anything that might in any way, violate care protocols. If in doubt, ask enough to know.

You may notice that I put nurses first in the asking chain of events. Nurses are key decision makers in care as they may often be more accessible and better equipped to do the detailed steps in a procedure.

You might think that Doctors' have more skill in doing a task and that is likely real but Time of intervention is critical in the

8

care of some patients, but nurses may have standing orders that allow them to act quickly. The doctors have the authority to work independently, which allows for more interventions.

While doctors manage patient care, you may notice that nurses, especially Triage Nurses, manage the priority order of care performance, so the doctors avoid the fragmentation of their focus.

Nurses work as part of the health care team, and they have their critical time priorities and intervention capabilities. Team structure allows an orchestrated alignment, so the doctors and nurses operate in a symphony of healing harmony.

Nurses greatly enhance the effectiveness of doctors and facilitate their ability to handle more patients expediently.

Like an orchestra, the music of healing needs the conductor and the full ensemble with all participants in optimal communication.

They are all balancing proficiency and speed, which is essential to doctors and nurses alike. While each group has skills that overlap, productivity and specialization allow the best results from the most adept skills of each with the least stress for all.

Teaching can be time intensive, so teaching patients may be more comfortable and more productive for all if the nurses teach the step by step protocols to patients, so there is a bit of extra time for the doctors to do oversight.

4 - Fear of Cancer Versus The Disease

The fear of Cancer is like a toxic waste as it can provide an environment that nurtures problem initiation and expansion. Fear can grab you consciously and subconsciously.

Fear and worry are pure trouble potentials. Together they make a terrible pair of pitfalls you could avoid. Consider each of them like a landmine that offer no good and could get you in more trouble.

Fear creates a kind of Mental block which can get in the way of you understanding the initiatives that you can bring into your life that align with a healing Path.

I wrote a blogpost about breaking up mental blocks, and it may help you break yours. The post is at the website of the Awaken Center For Human Evolution. The Direct Blog page is https://www.awakenche.org/blog/mental-energy-block-chops-6684

Worry may proceed or go along with fear. It is also something that you are best to eliminate. I wrote a book about stifling all worry.

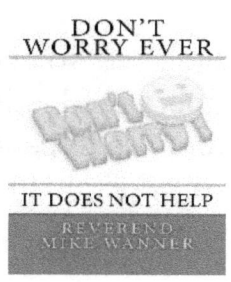

DON'T
WORRY EVER

IT DOES NOT HELP

REVEREND
MIKE WANNER

5 - Four Areas To Consider

There are Four support areas of our lives that we can work to keep in balance. They are:

> Physical Support
> Emotional Support
> Mental Support
> Spiritual Support

Each of these areas is significant because they all interact on an ongoing basis, and if one loses lift, then the connected ones within you are tweaked, and that is not healthy. On the next pages, I will offer an example of a method below for each area that needs to be supported. Other Methods can be useful, and I invite you to establish a separate effort of discovery into each spot with an emphasis on those that need attention for any emotional struggle that is current within you at a given time.

Physical Support

Your primary care and specialty care providers now need to be your high priority focus. Please be sure to listen to all they say and decide wisely.

It may be awkward, but now is a time that your Physical support choices could be irritated by reactionary emotionality. It is critical that you get a great deal of support from people who you trust.

Avoiding the information that is hard to hear can easily lead you to conveniently not listen to what you hear so it is crucial to have an advocate with you during your appointments if possible to note all the doctors say so they can remind you of essential information that you consciously or subconsciously deny hearing.

Information is a commodity that can significantly influence your ability to rearrange your life to enhance remedial tweaks.
Denying the depth of the problem helps nothing, but learning the details allows an optimal management and survival plan.

Emotional Support Systems

I have written a lot about Emotional Support in Ten earlier Cancer books which are also in two compendiums which include five of the titles each. All the books are in Chapter 14.

An energy modality called Integrated Energy Therapy has changed my life. It allows one to invoke Angelic energy for the release of stuffed emotions and cellular memory.

Integrated Energy Therapy can be used in person or sent at a distance to the one needing it. I am excited to think about using it along with or after Pranic Healing.

Mental Support System

Our minds can be our most reliable ally or our weakest link. When we allow our minds just to run, there seems to be a great cloud of possibilities on a scale from good to evil. When we take charge of our thoughts and direct them to a focus, then we can move toward a goal. Sorting through the many questions can be daunting.

The best resource that I have found so far is an ancient system called Dowsing that allows me to quickly run through possibilities and objectively help clients find goals that resonate with a progressive path out of an apparent state of overwhelming emotional paralysis.

Dowsing can be done in person or at a distance. There is a book on mine on it on the Cancer books by Mike page. I am excited to think about you using it along with or after Pranic Healing.

Powerful Quote About Intelligence

"An intelligent person is not closed-minded. He does not behave like an ostrich burying his head in the ground, trying to avoid new ideas and developments.

An intelligent person is not gullible. He does not accept ideas blindly.

He studies and digests them thoroughly, then evaluates them against his reason: he tests these new ideas and developments through experiments and his experiences.

An Intelligent person studies these ideas with a clear objective mind.

Shared by *Master Choa Kok Sui*

Spiritual Support Systems

I have also written a lot about Spiritual Support along with Emotional Support in earlier books that I compiled into two Compendiums, which include five of the titles each. A list of all the books is in Chapter 14.

Prayer is Powerful, and it's ability is increased with frequency. The frequency can be in that the person saying the prayer says more of them or the one who needs them can get the assistance of a person of prayer, a minister, a prayer circle, a prayer therapist or an on-line distant healing group to add to the efforts of the primary prayer.

One resource for prayer preciseness support is the webpage www.Create-A-Prayer.com. Prayer can be practiced in person or at a distance.

6 - Your Thinking Impacts Your Energy

Personal Power Declarations impact your energy profoundly. The following declarations are from Chapter 3, 3-1, 3-2, 3-3, 3-4, and 3-5 of the book Deep Daily Declarations: Personal Peace Brings Confidence. Confidence Helps Healing.

I Can Release Negativity

Worry Is a Waste of Time! I Can Stop doing It!

Worry Doesn't Help – Prayer Still Does!

Fear Is an Invitation From the Dark Side!
I Can Stop Being Fearful!

Hate is Toxic Self-Administered Poison!
Hate For Others May Be Personal or referred! Bad
Either Way. I Can Stop doing It! I Only Need To Fear
The Loss of God – Not God!

The Path Out of Darkness Is An Invitation like a prayer
– Lord Be With Me!

7 - Life Energy And The Breath

Living people and things depend on breathing. Without the breath, live ceases.

Air is essential as is the quality of that air. When a person is living in a contaminated environment, their life length can be short.

Every effort should be taken to have air that is as fresh and pure as possible.

The energy of our bodies, our life force is continually diminishing as we do things and apply motion to our muscles. The simple act of breathing uses the breath to breathe in new vibrancy.

While breathing and the life force or prana that it brings is very natural if not automatic during our youth, many things can happen to humans that influence our ability to breathe and create life force. Diminishing of our life force can also decrease our ability to reach an optimal age.

8 - Energy Systems Or Pranic Healing?

Before experiencing Pranic Healing, I imagined it as another healing energy system like many I have learned. When I experienced a little demo session during an Open House at The Awaken Center for Human Evolution (AwakenCHE.org), I was immediately impressed with the energy shift that I felt right after closing my eyes.

I scheduled a session to see if it was a one-off experience or whether there was more for me to feel. Again, I was immediately impressed and amazed.

If you ever told me that at the age of 74 that I would be racing to take new training, I would have said you were nuts. Well, Pranic Healing got my attention, and I booked the training and took it in short order.

Again I was impressed and amazed. I am sharing my impression because my experience is limited, and I recommend that readers do their investigation and evaluations.

If readers have their familiarity with other energy systems, then you have a base of comparison. If readers do not, then, I would recommend and have recommended energy work as nurture for those in a medical crisis or at a decision point.

In both the back of an ambulance and while ministering at the bedside, I have consistently had Cancer patients tell me about their insufficient energy so I suggest that all who can learn how to improve theirs, do so.

9 - Pranic Healing Has A Special Meditation

The Meditation for Pranic Healing is called the Meditation of the Twin Hearts.

It is declared as "… an integral part of pranic healing and is said to provide the strength the body needs to fight off infections, as well as helping practitioners learn to control their emotions and feel less anger, anxiety, and irritation, reduce stress, and improve concentration.

This type of meditation allows positive energy to flow through your body, which releases all of the negative energy. Scientific testing has shown people who practice meditation are healthier and more at peace mentally compared to others."

If you find the opportunity to tune-in to a performance of the meditation, I encourage you to give it a go.

Research News

Pranic Healing Research Institute reported that New research finds Meditation on Twin Hearts amplifies positive emotional regulation (Announcement dated March 31, 2019)

"Congratulations to Camila P. R. A. T. Valim, Lucas M. Marques and Paulo S. Boggio on their latest article *A Positive Emotional-Based Meditation but Not Mindfulness-Based Meditation Improves Emotion Regulation* published in *Frontiers in Psychology*, the world's most-cited multidisciplinary psychology journal.

The authors investigated the effect of meditation on the cognitive ability of emotion regulation, comparing Meditation on Twin Hearts and mindfulness meditation. The participants who practiced a single Meditation on Twin Hearts were more effective in suppressing negative emotion and amplifying positive emotion than those who practiced mindfulness meditation and the control group."

10 - Simplified Beginning Ideas

If you or someone you care about is in an illness crisis, resources can be sparse. While many things could offer some promise, it may be challenging to figure out the optimal ones for the needs of the person you want to help.

If you can get access to a book on Pranic Healing, you can begin to educate yourself and take one step at a time.

I particularly like the book "Miracles Through Pranic Healing." It is on kindle for $13.99. When you start that book even before you get to Chapter One, there are pages titled " How To Practice Simplified Pranic Healing Immediately."

A feature of the Pranic Healing Process is the use of precise step-by-step instructions, a kind of recipe for a healing process. While this Simplified Pranic Healing procedure can be a demonstration of effectiveness, it is not as applicable to all potential challenges as the full system.

There are twelve steps in the procedure that are to go in sequence. Eleven of those steps are to read the specific text, and the twelfth is to do a treatment that could last 20 minutes to an hour.

The first eleven steps are described as readable within a time frame of two hours. The eleven steps are:

1. Learn about the eleven essential chakras.
2. Practice connecting the tongue to the roof of the mouth,

3. Read about the procedure process for Bioplasmic waste disposal.
4. Review General sweeping technique.
5. Review the Localized sweeping technique.
6. Learn about Diseased Energy Contamination &.Handwashing Techniques.
7. Patient Receptivity assistance.
8. Energizing with Prana & Hand Chakra Technique.
9. Stabilizing the Projected Prana
10. Releasing the Projected Prana
11. Five things to avoid in Pranic Healing

The 12th step is Pranic Treatment for 20 minutes to an hour. I Recommend that you consider that and all the steps above as an investment in your wellness.

Pranic Healing Resources Local to You?

I would encourage you to visit the websites - *www.pranichealingusa.com* & *www.pranichealingpenn.com* and https://www.meetup.com/Pranic-Healing-Bucks-County-Meetup/ and network amongst spiritual healing, holistic, and wellness organizations to see what resources you can find. :

Look for Open Heart Meditations, Pranic Healing Demos, Pranic Healing Practitioners (Try a Treatment), Holistic Venues & Body Mind & Spirit Events, Naturopaths, Chiropractors, etc.

11 - Wrap Up

I hope this book allows more people to find options for the healing they and their families need.

There are some high potentials to be had with the energy work of many modalities.

The significant factor in pranic healing that I like is the Energy Cleaning, which is akin to smoothing out existing energy and removing some negative energy to clear the way for fresh infusions of subtle energy.

May all who read these words have their energy increase, AND SO IT IS! Amen and Amen!

12 - A Place To Start Learning

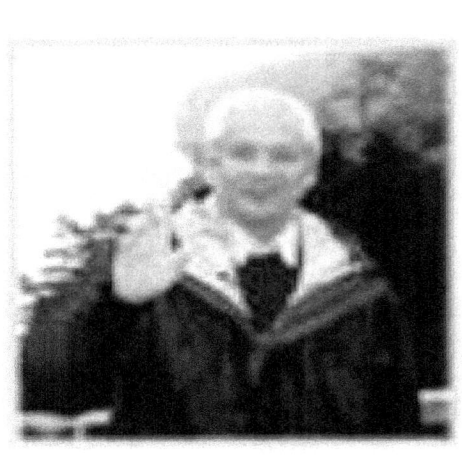

The Origin of Modern Pranic Healing and Arhatic Yoga Master Choa Kok Sui by Master Choa Kok Sui

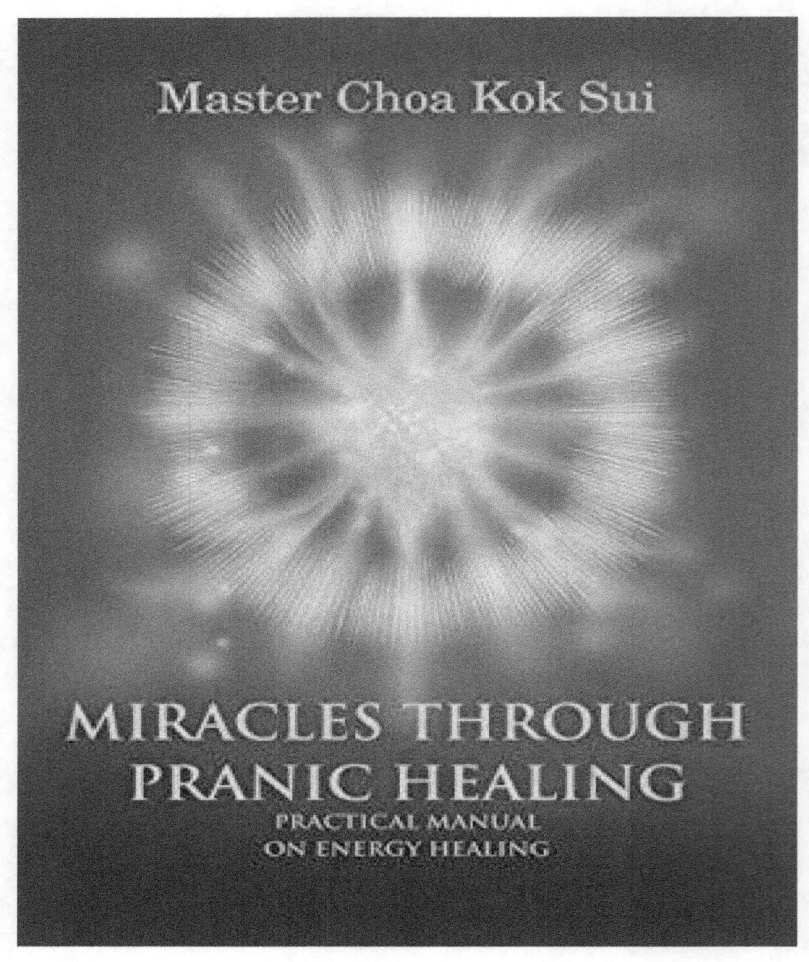

Miracles Through Pranic Healing
by Master Choa Kok Sui

24

"This book is more than brilliant—it is essential for all readers who value the quality of their health."
—CAROLINE MYSS, AUTHOR OF SACRED CONTRACTS

YOUR HANDS CAN HEAL YOU

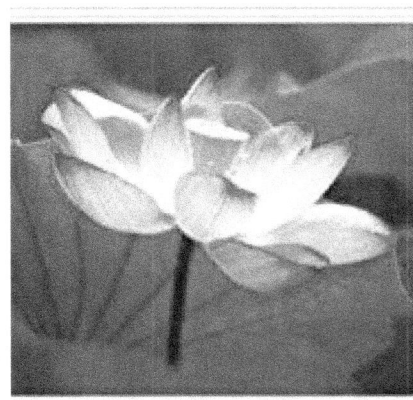

PRANIC HEALING
ENERGY REMEDIES
TO BOOST VITALITY
AND SPEED RECOVERY
FROM COMMON
HEALTH PROBLEMS

MASTER STEPHEN CO &
ERIC B. ROBINS, M.D.
WITH JOHN MERRYMAN

Your Hands Can Heal You: Pranic Healing Energy Remedies to Boost
Vitality and Speed Recovery from Common Health Problems
by Master Stephen Co, Eric B. Robins

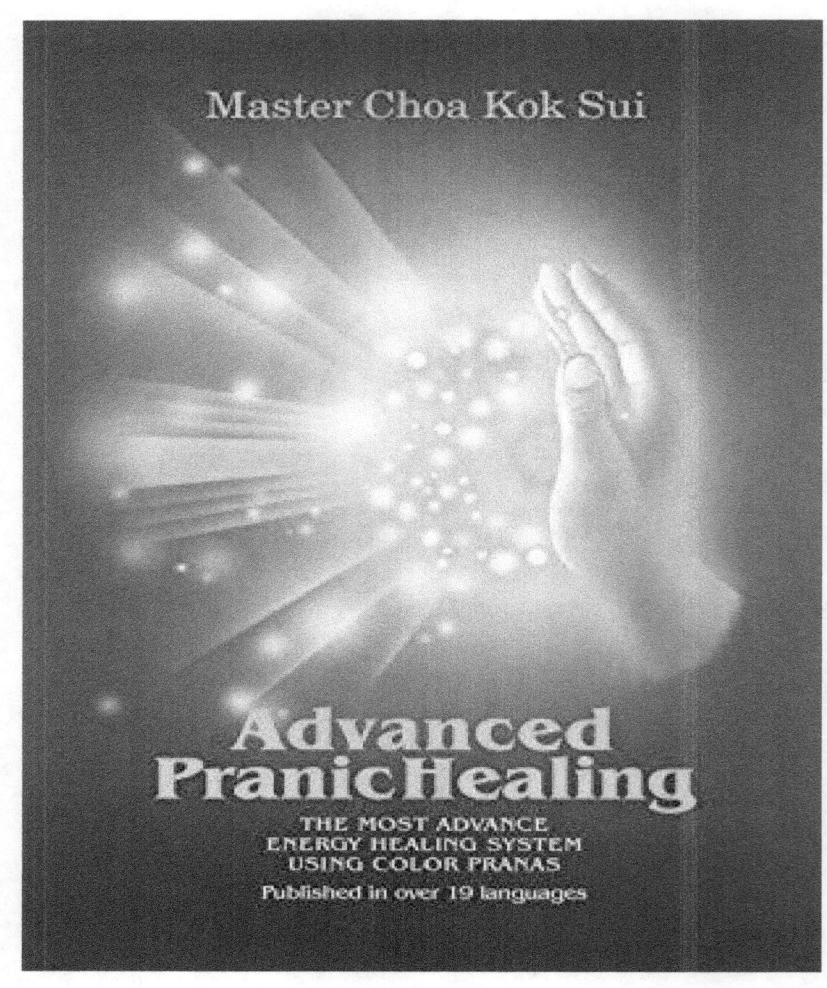

Advanced Pranic Healing
by Master Choa Kok Sui

26

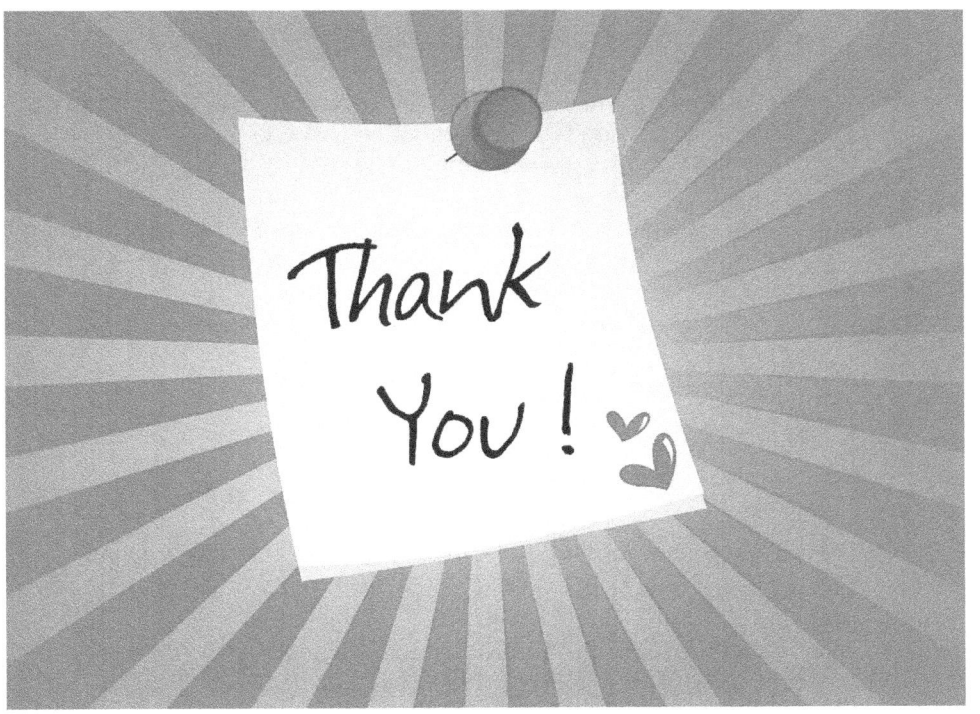

For
Considering
These
Ideas

14 - Other Cancer Books by Rev. Mike

Cancer Emotional And Spiritual Compendium: Caring To Support Cancer Care
http://amzn.com/B07N9XYF9R

Cancer Emotional And Spiritual Compendium Volume Two: Caring From An Earlier Time Plus Recent & New Books
http://amzn.com/B07RZD37TM

Does Reiki Love Heal Cancer?: Transcribed True Stories Of Spiritual Healing
http://amzn.com/B00MS6M77I

Reiki Help For Cancer Care in Pottstown, PA: Cecilia Appreciates PMMC Cancer Center
http://amzn.com/B071XBTSFX

Reiki For Cancer
http://amzn.com/B07873YKLJ

Love Energy Circuit Healing For Cancer Patients: Energize & Bond
http://amzn.com/B07QPWGXM1

Cancer Patient's Self-Talk And Reflections: Think High Vibration!
http://amzn.com/B07R7YLNWR

Cancer Glue For Adults: Love From Kids
http://amzn.com/B07JMK6FWG

Cancer Glue For Adults: Love From Reiki
http://amzn.com/B07JQPBWW6

Cancer Glue For You: Family Energy
http://amzn.com/B07KM92DMD

Cancer Glue For Miracles: Believing & Preparing & Expecting
http://amzn.com/B07MHK4XZ2

Cancer Glue For Possibilities: Dowsing Power
http://amzn.com/B07M74L8DV

15 - Books Category Resources
at www.Amazon.com

Distant Healing (or Mail List) e-mail mikewann@voicenet.com

Veterans Healing Six Pack plus 2
http://angelraphaelspeaks.com/healing-books/veterans/

PTSD Power Pack
http://angelraphaelspeaks.com/healing-books/ptsd/

Angel Raphael Speaks Series & Other Angel Books
http://angelraphaelspeaks.com/

Reiki
http://angelraphaelspeaks.com/healing-books/reiki/

Children
http://angelraphaelspeaks.com/healing-books/children/

Emergency Medical Kindness
http://angelraphaelspeaks.com/healing-books/emergency-medical-kindness/

Cancer
http://angelraphaelspeaks.com/healing-books/cancer/

Addictions
http://angelraphaelspeaks.com/healing-books/addictions/

Miscellaneous Healing
http://angelraphaelspeaks.com/healing-books/misc-healing/

Prison Books - 60+ Prison Books
http://angelraphaelspeaks.com/prison-books/

16 - Angels Please Prayers For Addiction

Addict's
Angels of Healing Selected
Help Me to Stay Directed
Come To Me From The Sky
I Am Ready to Succeed Not Try
If I Don't Invite You In
I Might Not Win
I Have Been Lost For Too Long
Help Me To Stay Strong

Alcoholic's
Angels of Healing On High
Help Me to Stay Dry
Come To Me From The Sky
I Am Ready to Succeed Not Try
If I Don't Invite You In
I Might Not Win
I Have Been Lost For Too Long
Help Me To Stay Strong

Prayers Above From

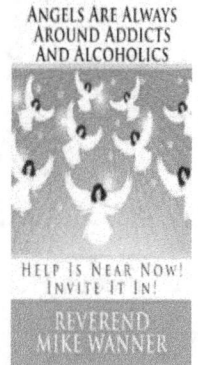

http://AngelRaphaelSpeaks.com/AAAAAAA/
The Link Above Has the Core Messages from the book on drop-down pages.

17 - Private Channeling

Angel Raphael Speaks is a series of free messages channeled through Reverend Mike Wanner for the Highest good and Highest Healing of all concerned.

Many questions arise about Reverend Mike doing private channeling, and he does help with that so E-mail him.

Reverend Mike is available worldwide as a psychic channel, emotional release facilitator, spiritual energy practitioner & teacher, and public speaker.

He looks forward to meeting you soon! Email - mikewann@voicenet.com 215-342-1270

PRIVATE SPIRITUAL READINGS/channelings or Spiritual Healing Sessions can be by Telephone or in person.

Rev. Mike is available for individual, intuitive one-on-one sessions with you, his Guide Family, and your Guides. He helps by offering clarity on emotional situations about your life, your purpose, your spirituality, and your release of stuffed emotions and cellular memory.

Connect to the love of your Guides today!

For more information, Please visit
http://angelraphaelspeaks.com/channel/

18 - Reverend Mike Wanner

Rev. Mike Wanner started his spiritual and ministerial studies with Reiki in 1993 and had studied seven styles of Reiki in the U.S., Japan, Canada, Denmark, and Australia. He is certified to teach.

He became certified to teach Integrated Energy Therapy in 1999 and co-taught the first IET class of the new Millennium. Mike began dowsing in 2001.

Ordained as an Interfaith Minister of the Circle of Miracles Ministry and a Metaphysical Minister of the International Metaphysical Ministry, Rev. Mike practices and teaches spiritual energy therapies in the Philadelphia Area.

Rev. Mike holds ministerial degrees from the University of Metaphysics and the University of Sedona. He is a Pastoral Care Associate at Jefferson - Frankford Hospital. He taught at the National Academy of Massage Therapy and Health Sciences.

Rev. Mike was a faculty member of the Medical Mission Sister's Center for Human Integration's School of Integrated Body/Mind Therapies in Fox Chase, Philadelphia, PA, for twelve years.

For a complete Biography, Please visit
http://ReverendMikeWanner.com/Bio

www.ingramcontent.com/pod-product-compliance
Lightning Source LLC
Chambersburg PA
CBHW071445170526
45158CB00005BA/1842